"Dr. Robert Shipley, director of the prestigious Duke University Quit Smoking Clinic, has come up with a tool to help people through the struggle... The appealing prose, cartoons and charts make for engaging reading."

Mark J. Tager, M.D.
American Journal of Health Promotion

"Advice on how to quit smoking is easy to come by. This book, however, is considerably more than mere advice. It represents the results of many years of research on methods for successful quitting."

Patrick A. Boudewyns, Ph.D.
Professor, Department of Psychiatry
  and Health Behavior
Medical College of Georgia

"A remarkably clear, practical guide to assist those who want to stop smoking!"

John R. Feussner, M.D.
Director, Center for Health Services
  Research in Primary Care
Department of Veterans Affairs

"The QuitSmart book and CD are terrific. It is the finest, most useful tool I've ever seen to help smokers quit. I'm recommending it to all my patients who are smokers."

Belinda R. Novik, Ph.D.
Practicing Clinical Psychologist
Past President, North Carolina Society
  of Clinical Hypnosis

"The QuitSmart Stop Smoking Kit is easy to use, interactive, and informative... I enthusiastically recommend the kit."

Crystal L. Dunlevy, Ed.D., RRT
Respiratory Care Journal

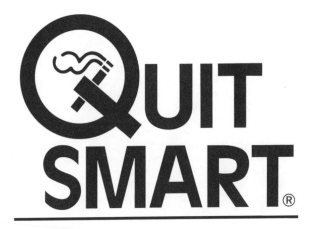

STOP SMOKING GUIDE

It's easier than you think

Dr. Robert H. Shipley

QuitSmart Stop Smoking Resources, Inc., P.O. Box 99016,
Duke Station, Durham, NC 27708-9016, 888-737-6278 or
919-644-6522. For ordering information, turn to the last page
of this guide or go to www.QuitSmart.com.

ISBN numbers:

1-880781-09-3	2009 QuitSmart Stop Smoking Guidebook
1-880781-08-5	2009 QuitSmart Stop Smoking Kit (QuitSmart Guidebook, Hypnosis CD, and Cigarette Substitute)

Special thanks to: Dr. Jed Rose for information on
pre-cessation use of the nicotine patch, Dr. Jonathan Foulds
for comments on the medication sections of this book, and
Dr. Alice White and Susan Tanner for editing and design help.

Cover design by Jamie Sanders

Typesetting by Deidra Stierle

Printed in the United States of America

To the thousands of exsmokers who allowed me to share their journey,

and

to Alice, Kimra, Jennifer, Kendall, Spud, Major, and our Scottie, Piper.

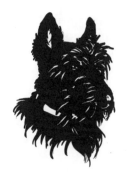

PREFACE

I'm excited about this revision of the QuitSmart Guidebook. The previous editions were good—three studies show double or triple the quit rates of other methods—but this one's better!

It shows how you can safely start the nicotine patch *before* you quit, and dramatically increase your chance of success. And you'll see how to really control cigarette cravings by using the nicotine lozenge or gum in addition to the nicotine patch. You'll also discover new ways to overcome the habit of smoking.

Mixed feelings are normal. I've been helping people break free from cigarettes for a long time. I know you want to quit smoking. You want to breathe easier, have more energy, and not worry about the sickness and early death that smoking often brings.

I know too that part of you enjoys smoking, and that you worry you won't be able to cope without cigarettes. You may also fear the quitting process: the cravings, withdrawal symptoms, and possibility of failure. These are common concerns, but there are now so many tools to help you.

You can succeed with QuitSmart. It takes a firm decision to quit, and a determination to use the coping methods taught in this guidebook. Brand-switching, stop-smoking medicine, and hypnosis are some of the tools you'll use to break free from cigarettes for good.

This is personal for me. I used to smoke. I've had cancer. My father, a smoker, died of a heart attack at age 64. He's not alone—smoking causes an early death in one of every two long-term smokers. I don't like those odds. I want you to live a long, healthy life.

You can QuitSmart!
Bob Shipley

CONTENTS

INTRODUCTION

Congratulations on taking the first step to break free from cigarettes by reading this guidebook. You will learn proven ways to quit.

It's most important that you make a *firm* decision to quit. Then use the coping methods and medicines suggested in this guidebook to make your decision a reality.

You will learn how to:

- Reduce your nicotine intake by gradually switching to low-nicotine cigarettes.

- Use stop-smoking medicines to reduce cravings and withdrawal symptoms.

- Use your thoughts to make quitting easier.

- Use hypnosis to relax and focus on success.

- Avoid smoking temptations and come-ons.

- Use a fake cigarette to cope with your hand-to-mouth habit.

- Get the right kind of support from family and friends.

- Control your weight.

- Add pleasures to offset the loss of smoking.

Using this Guidebook

This guide has a chapter on each phase of quitting:

1. Preparing to Quit
2. Quitting
3. Remaining a Nonsmoker

During each phase, study the chapter for that phase and for the next one. For example, after reading Chapter 1 (*Preparing to Quit*), read Chapter 2 (*Quitting*). That way you'll be prepared for what's ahead.

Carry this guidebook with you and refer to it often. Practice the suggested coping methods, even if some seem a bit silly or unneeded. By using the methods in this guide, you have a very good chance of success.

Smokeless Tobacco

This guidebook is focused on cigarette smokers. However, most of the recommended coping methods and medicines also apply to users of snuff and chewing tobacco. Two methods to help snuff users reduce nicotine intake are presented on page 21.

Smokeless tobacco is not a safe substitute for cigarettes. It can cause oral cancer, pancreatic cancer, gum disease, tooth loss, and high blood pressure.

www.killthecan.org

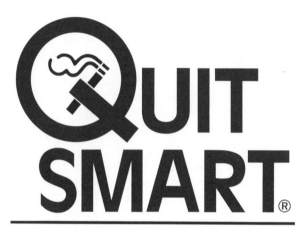

CHAPTER 1
Preparing to Quit

Just as you plan for a trip by thinking ahead and deciding what to take along, this chapter will help you prepare to quit. There are five essential steps:

Focus on your reasons for quitting. This will help you understand that you are quitting for you, not for someone else.

Reduce your nicotine intake. Before you quit, gradually switch to lower-nicotine cigarettes.

Use stop-smoking medicine. It's a smart way to control smoking urges, lessen withdrawal symptoms, and increase your chance of quitting.

Create a supportive environment. Ask family and friends for help and smoke proof your home and workplace.

Make a firm decision to quit. This is the time to resolve ambivalence and set a firm quit date.

REASONS FOR QUITTING

It can be difficult to decide to quit smoking because so many people are pushing you to quit. Pressure may be coming from your family, friends, employers, and doctors.

Ignore the pressure. No one can make you quit. In fact, pressure can backfire, causing you to dig in your heels and think, "Those anti-smokers can't make me quit."

The decision to quit must be yours, based on your own reasons. After all, you are the one who will do the work to quit, and who will give up the pleasure of smoking. Other people's reasons don't matter much.

Take control. You may have started to smoke, in part, to show that you were an adult who could do whatever you wanted. But are you still in control, or are cigarettes controlling you? Breaking free from cigarettes puts you in control.

List your reasons. Put a check mark by each reason on the next page that matches your own. Write in your unique reasons below the list. Use the list as a reminder of why *you* decided to break free from cigarettes.

I am quitting so:

- [x] I will not have to worry so much about cancer, heart disease, and stroke.

- [x] I will breathe easier.

- [ ] My skin will look healthier.

- [ ] I will have fewer colds and less congestion.

- [x] I will have more energy.

- [ ] I will not feel like a social outcast.

- [ ] I will stop coughing.

- [ ] My children and grandchildren will be protected from secondhand smoke.

- [ ] I will no longer worry about starting an accidental fire.

- [x] I will wake up feeling more rested.

- [ ] I will smell better to others.

- [ ] My sour stomach will improve.

- [x] My house and car will be cleaner.

- [ ] My teeth will be whiter.

- [ ] My sports performance will improve.

- [x] I will save lots of money.

- [ ] I will feel more in control of my life.

- [x] My wife, an ex-smoker, doesn't
- [ ] have temptation around.
- [ ] _____

Before you quit, reduce your nicotine intake by gradually switching to brands of cigarettes that deliver less and less nicotine. We call this *Warm Chicken* quitting. It's easier than quitting cold turkey.

Find your brand's nicotine rating. Find the nicotine rating of your cigarette brand by locating it in the boxes on the following pages. For example, if you smoke Marlboro Full Flavor, each cigarette is rated at 1.1 milligrams nicotine (Box 11). Other Marlboro brands (Lights and Ultra-Lights) have different nicotine ratings, so be sure to find your exact brand.

Select your new brands. Inside the box listing your cigarette brand are instructions to switch to a new box. Select a brand from the new box and smoke it for seven days. Then choose a brand from the next indicated box, and smoke it for seven days. If you originally smoked an average-nicotine brand (Boxes 6–10), two brand switches will complete the procedure.

If you smoked a high-nicotine brand (Boxes 11–17), you will need to switch brands three times. Switches are made every seven days so this will take three weeks. However, if you are in a QuitSmart class, you will be asked to switch brands every 4–5 days so you can finish in time for the class quit date in two weeks.

Example. Gerry smoked thirty Basic Full Flavor cigarettes a day. She found this brand in Box 10 and saw that she should switch to a brand in Box 4. She selected Winston Ultra-Lights and smoked thirty of these a day for one week. For the second week she switched to Carlton Kings in Box 2. Then she quit, with few withdrawal symptoms.

Be sure you actually get less nicotine. In smoking each new brand, be careful not to smoke more cigarettes than usual or to inhale more deeply. Also, avoid blocking the tiny holes around the filter of many cigarettes— these holes draw in fresh air and lower nicotine intake. Your lips should not cover more than ½ inch of the filter end, and your fingers should not be on the filter.

Why not just smoke less? Reducing nicotine intake by smoking fewer cigarettes does not help most people quit. As you cut back the number of cigarettes, each remaining cigarette becomes more pleasurable. It is very difficult to give up the last few. On the other hand, when you switch to very low-nicotine brands, each cigarette is a bit unpleasant and giving them up is much easier.

One switch with pre-quit nicotine patch. A new option for nicotine patches is to begin using them two weeks *before* your quit date (p. 30–31). In that case, you make only one brand switch directly to very low-nicotine cigarettes.

CIGARETTE NICOTINE RATINGS

In this section, cigarette brands are grouped from high to low nicotine rating. Begin by finding your exact brand in one of the boxes. Below the blue bar in the box, you'll see *Switch next to Box...* Select a brand from that box to smoke over the next week. Continue to switch brands each week. Quit after you complete Box 2.

Brand labels. Brands in the boxes may be Full Flavor (FF), Light (L), or Ultra-Light (U-Lt). All are filtered unless listed as non-filter (NF). Unless otherwise specified, each brand's nicotine rating applies to menthol and non-menthol and to all sizes of that brand (kings, 100s, & 120s).

Can't find your brand? Your brand may not be listed if it is a new brand or a low-price brand. Follow these guidelines to estimate your brand's nicotine rating:

Non-filter	➡	1.5 mg (Box 15)
Filter		
Full Flavor	➡	1.0 mg (Box 10)
Light	➡	0.8 mg (Box 8)
Ultra-Light	➡	0.5 mg (Box 4)

Machine versus smoker. The nicotine values listed here were determined by a smoking machine. Real smokers get about twice as much nicotine. The machine values, while not perfect, allow us to rank brands from high to low nicotine delivery.

17   1.7 Milligrams Nicotine or More

Switch next to Box 9

Camel NF
Doral NF
Grand Prix NF
Liggett Select NF

Natural American Spirit
Natural Am. Spirit NF
Pyramid NF

15   1.5–1.6 Milligrams Nicotine

Switch next to Box 8

Class A NF
Grand Prix NF
Liggett Select NF

Max 120s
Newport FF
Pall Mall NF

13   1.3–1.4 Milligrams Nicotine

Switch next to Box 8

Camel FF
Chesterfield NF
English Ovals NF
Kamel Red
Kool FF
Lucky Strike NF

Maverick 100s
Natural Am. Spirit Lt.
Old Gold FF
Pall Mall FF
Salem FF
Seneca FF

12   1.2 Milligrams Nicotine

Switch next to Box 6

Basic NF
Camel Turkish FF
Commander NF
GPC NF
Kent 100s

Monarch NF
Newport Medium
Players Navy Cut NF
Winston FF
Winston Select FF

11   1.1 Milligrams Nicotine

Switch next to Box 6

Benson & Hedges FF
Camel #9 FF
Chesterfield FF
Eve 120s Lt
Marlboro FF
Maverick Kings

More
Newport Lt 100s
Parliament FF
Saratoga 120s
Virginia Slims FF
Virginia Slims Luxury Lt

10   1.0 Milligrams Nicotine

Switch next to Box 4

Basic FF
Doral FF
Cambridge FF
Capri
Class A FF
Daves FF
Grand Prix FF
Kent Kings
Kool Mild
L & M FF
Lark FF

Liggett Select FF
Lucky Strike FF
Misty Slim 120s Lt
Natural American Spirit
  Organic Lt
Pall Mall Lt
Parliament 100s Lt
Pyramid FF
Seneca Lt
USA FF

9 0.9 Milligrams Nicotine

Switch next to Box 4

Benson & Hedges Multifilter
Camel Lt
GPC FF
Kamel Red Lt
Kent Lt
Kent Golden Lt
Marlboro Blend 27
Marlboro Medium
Marlboro Milds

Monarch FF
More Lt
Pall Mall Gold
Tareyton FF
Winston Lt
Winston Select Lt
Winston Slim Lt
Winston S2

8 0.8 Milligrams Nicotine

Switch next to Box 4

Basic Lt
Benson & Hedges Lt
Camel #9 Lt
Camel Turkish Lt/Gold/Silver
Capri Lt
Chesterfield Lt
Class A Lt
GPC Lt
Grand Prix Lt
Kool Lt
Lark Lt

Liggett Select Lt
Lucky Strike Lt
Marlboro Lt
Newport Lt Kings
Old Gold Lt
Pyramid Lt
Salem Lt
Seneca U-Lt
USA Lt
Vantage

Remember, for each brand, the nicotine rating listed applies to all lengths of that brand (kings, 100s, 120s) and to menthol and nonmenthol varieties (unless otherwise specified).

6   0.6–0.7 Milligrams Nicotine

Switch next to Box 4

Cambridge Lt
Capri U-Lt
Davies Lt
Doral Lt
Eve 120s U-Lt
GPC Lt
Kent III U-Lt
L&M Lt
Merit Lt
Misty 100s Lt

Monarch Lt
Montego U-Lt
Natrual Am Spirit U-Lt
Pall Mall U-Lt
Parliament Kings Lt
Quest 1
True 100s
Virginia Slims Lt
Virginia SuperSlims

4   0.3–0.5 Milligrams Nicotine

Switch next to Box 2

Benson & Hedges U-Lt
Cambridge U-Lt
Camel U-Lt
Carlton 120s
Class A U-Lt
Doral U-Lt
Grand Prix U-Lt
Liggett Select U-Lt
Marlboro U-Lt
Merit U-Lt
Misty Slim U-Lt
Monarch U-Lt

Now 100s
Old Gold U-Lt
Parliment U-Lt
Pyramid U-Lt
Quest 2
Salem U-Lt
True Kings
USA U-Lt
Vantage U-Lt
Virginia Slims U-Lt
Winston U-Lt

2   0.2 Milligrams Nicotine or Less

You are Ready to Quit

Carlton Kings   Merit Ultima
Carlton 100s   Now Kings

Snuff Users

Choose one of two ways to reduce nicotine intake before quitting: brand switching or herbal snuff tapering.

Brand switching. Switch each week to a snuff brand with less nicotine.

High nicotine: Copenhagen, Cougar Regular or LC Natural, Kodiak, Red Seal, Rooster, Skoal (except Cherry or Berry & Bandits), Timber Wolf Straight or Long Cut

Medium nicotine: Cougar LC Wintergreen, Skoal LC Cherry or Berry, Timber Wolf Fine Cut

Low nicotine: Hawken Wintergreen, Renegade, Skoal Bandits, Silver Creek

- OR -

Herbal snuff tapering. Mix your regular snuff with nicotine-free herbal snuff: Mix in ⅓ herbal snuff the first week, and ⅔ the second week. If you can't find herbal snuff, visit:

www.smokeysnuff.com
www.mintsnuff.com

There are seven stop-smoking medicines. The table below shows how long to use each medicine, the approximate cost, and the Success Multiplier—how much each multiplies your chance of success over trying to quit without using medicine.

Non-Prescription Medicines

Medicine	Months to Use	$/Month (generic)	Success Multiplier
Nicotine Patch	2–6	$80 (50)	2x
2 mg Nicotine Gum or Lozenge	3–6	$120 (95)	2x
4 mg Nicotine Gum or Lozenge	3–6	$120 (95)	3x

Prescription Medicines

Medicine	Months to Use	$/Month (generic)	Success Multiplier
Nicotine Nasal Spray	3–6	$115	2x
Nicotine Inhaler	3–6	$150	2x
Zyban (Bupropion ER)	2–6	$220 (30)	2x
Chantix	3–6	$160	3x

In the following pages you will learn more about each medicine, and discover two new ways to use these medicines.

- **Combine two medicines.** Use the nicotine patch plus another nicotine medicine, like the gum or lozenge, for a 3.5x Success Multiplier.

- **Use the patch before quitting.** Start the patch two weeks before quitting, and continue it after you quit. This multiplies your success chances 4x.

Check with Your Doctor

My advice on using stop-smoking medicine is based on my clinical experience, research studies, and the advice of other experts.

Sometimes this advice differs from that of the U.S. Food and Drug Administration (FDA) and the medicine's manufacturer. I cover some common side effects, but not all possible ones. Your doctor can discuss other precautions and possible medication interactions to be sure that you choose the best medicine(s) for you.

When you stop smoking, whether or not you use stop-smoking medicine, other medicines you take may be absorbed differently. Ask your doctor if the strength of your other medicines needs to be changed.

Temporary use of nicotine-replacement medicine relieves smoking urges, reduces withdrawal symptoms, and doubles or triples your chance of quitting success. Unfortunately, some people resist using nicotine medicine because they think it's addictive and dangerous.

Nicotine is highly addictive, right?

It depends on how fast the nicotine reaches your brain. A puff on a cigarette gives a pleasurable nicotine jolt in just ten seconds. This quick pleasure keeps you coming back for more—it's highly addictive.

Nicotine in medicine is delivered slowly. It takes 20 minutes for nicotine from the gum or lozenge to reach peak levels, from the patch it takes 3–4 hours. This slow nicotine reduces cravings and withdrawal symptoms without giving the quick pleasure that causes addiction.

Of course, a few people continue to use nicotine medicine for a long time and some believe they are addicted. However, the vast majority can ease off the medicine when they choose. Rather than using these medicines too long, many people stop too soon and risk a return to smoking.

Isn't nicotine dangerous?

Nicotine medicine is completely safe for most people, but check with your doctor if you are pregnant, diabetic, or have severe heart trouble.

Nicotine in cigarettes is dangerous because the quick hits keep you addicted, and smoking. Cigarette smoke contains a toxic stew of 4000 chemicals, including carbon monoxide, radioactive polonium-210, and hydrogen cyanide.

Is nicotine medicine expensive?

Compare the cost of nicotine medicine to what you spend on cigarettes. If you're smoking a pack a day at $5.00 a pack, that's $150 a month—every month, forever. Generic nicotine patches cost about $50 a month for as little as two months. Then you're free.

Can I use two nicotine medicines?

Yes, to get enough nicotine you may need to use both the patch and either the lozenge, gum, nasal spray, or inhaler. Use the added nicotine medicine every hour or two to raise your nicotine intake to a comfortable level. Plus, reach for more to relieve cravings.

How much nicotine medicine do I need?

Ideally you want at least as much nicotine from your medicine as you got from your cigarettes. However, it's difficult to determine how much nicotine you got from cigarettes.

Nicotine from cigarettes. The standard nicotine rating of each cigarette brand is determined by a smoking machine. The machine takes a small puff on a cigarette every 60 seconds. But most smokers take larger, more frequent puffs. When the machine is set to take a larger puff every 30 seconds, more like a real smoker, *nicotine ratings can double.*

Looking at Marlboro Full Flavor (FF) cigarettes, the nicotine rating goes from 1.1 mg nicotine when measured by the standard method, to 2.1 mg when measured by the more realistic method. The rating for Marlboro Lights increases from 0.8 mg to 1.6 mg nicotine.

An example. Frank smoked a pack-a-day of Marlboro FF cigarettes. He may need 42 mg of nicotine medicine to be comfortable because he likely was getting that much from his cigarettes (20 cigarettes x 2.1 mg nicotine per cigarette).

A 21 mg patch would replace only half the nicotine from Frank's cigarettes. This would help some, but probably would not be enough nicotine to keep him comfortable. Adding ten 4 mg lozenges would likely do the trick (only 2 mg of nicotine is absorbed from each "4 mg" lozenge).

Adjust your nicotine dose. Pay attention to how you feel and give yourself more or less nicotine medicine as needed. Just as you smoked more if you felt irritable, anxious, or had cigarette cravings, use more nicotine medicine if you have these feelings. Use less if you have symptoms, such as a queasy stomach, that would have led you to smoke less.

In the example above, if Frank started using 4 mg lozenges but soon felt dizzy or nauseous (signs of too much nicotine), he could use fewer

4 mg lozenges or switch to 2 mg lozenges. On the other hand, if Frank used ten 4 mg lozenges a day and still had cigarette cravings and withdrawal symptoms, he could use more lozenges.

What if I get too much nicotine?

If you have signs of too much nicotine— nausea, dizziness, cold sweat, fast or irregular heartbeat—cut back on the amount of nicotine medicine. If you don't feel better, stop using the medicine and call your doctor.

If I smoke should I stop the medicine?

No. If you slip up and smoke a cigarette, you are at high risk of going back to regular smoking. That is no time to be without nicotine medicine. Don't let the slip throw you. Keep using your nicotine medicine and resolve to stay completely smokefree.

How long should I stay on the medicine?

Use full-strength nicotine medicine for at least six weeks. Then, continue on this dose until you go 14 days in a row without strong cravings or withdrawal symptoms such as irritability or difficulty concentrating. Only then should you start *gradually* reducing your dose.

If you use the patch plus another nicotine medicine, wean off the patch first. Then gradually reduce your use of the other medicine. Even after you stop regular use, continue to carry some nicotine medicine to help with occasional cravings.

I often recommend the nicotine patch because it's easy to use, affordable, and available without a prescription. The patch takes the edge off cravings, and reduces anxiety, irritability, and difficulty concentrating.

Because the patch provides a steady level of nicotine, it is a good choice if you smoke throughout the day. If you smoke only at certain times of the day, a better choice may be the nicotine lozenge, gum, inhaler, or nasal spray.

How do I use the patch?

Apply a new patch to your skin every morning, starting on your quit date. Place the patch on an area that is dry, relatively hairless, and free of moisturizer from lotion or soap. Possible places include the upper arms, thighs, stomach, back, and chest. Press around the edges of the patch so it sticks well.

The skin under the patch may itch, tingle, or feel warm for up to an hour. When you remove the patch, the skin may be irritated. If so, don't use that spot again for at least a week.

Should I leave the patch on overnight?

For the best control of morning cravings, leave the patch on overnight. However, if you have difficulty falling asleep or have vivid dreams, take the patch off an hour before bedtime. When you apply a new patch the next morning, it will take several hours for nicotine to build up in your system—during that time, consider using nicotine gum, lozenges, inhaler, or nasal spray.

What strength patch should I use?

Most patches come in three strengths: 21 mg, 14 mg, and 7 mg. If you smoked

- 11 or more cigarettes a day, start on the strongest patch (21 mg).

- 10 or fewer cigarettes a day, start on the middle-strength patch (14 mg).

Will I get the right amount of nicotine?

You likely are getting less nicotine than you need if you have strong urges to smoke, or feel irritable, restless, drowsy, or sad. If you're already using the strongest patch, add a second nicotine medicine like nicotine gum or lozenges (unless your doctor objects).

On the other hand, if you think you are getting too much nicotine, switch to a weaker patch. If you don't feel better over several hours, remove the patch and check with your doctor.

How long should I use the patch?

Stay on your original-strength patch at least six weeks, and until you have gone 14 days in a row without strong cravings or withdrawal symptoms. Only then start to step down to weaker patches.

www.nicodermcq.com

Starting the patch on your quit date doubles your chance of quitting, a Success Multiplier of 2x. Now studies show that starting the patch two weeks *before* you quit, and continuing it afterward, gives a Success Multiplier of 4x!

Is it safe?

Recent studies find little danger from smoking while using patches, though the label on patches in the U.S. still warns against it. Australia has approved pre-quit use of the patch and fourteen other countries approve using various nicotine medicines while the user continues to smoke.

How does it help?

Wearing the patch while you are smoking weakens the link between smoking and pleasure. Usually when you smoke, each puff on a cigarette feeds your nicotine-starved brain. When you wear a patch your brain already has nicotine, so smoking doesn't give you much pleasure. It's like eating a meal when you're already full.

Switch to low-nicotine cigarettes

When you start using the patch, switch to very low-nicotine cigarettes. That will keep you from getting more nicotine than you're used to. The switch to low-nicotine cigarettes may also increase your chance of quitting success.

How do I use this strategy?

If you usually smoke 11 or more cigarettes a day, start on the strongest patch two weeks before your quit date. If you smoke 10 or fewer cigarettes a day, do not use the patch before you quit.

When you start on the patch, switch to a very-low nicotine cigarette brand from Box 2, page 21. Don't go through the whole brand-switching routine—go directly to a very low nicotine brand. Smoke your usual number of cigarettes unless you need to smoke fewer to avoid symptoms of too much nicotine (nausea, dizziness, fast or irregular heartbeat).

Use the patch as described on page 28. After your quit date, continue to use the patch and add another nicotine medicine if needed.

Precautions

- Check with your doctor about pre-quit patch use. Share information in this guidebook and refer your doctor to: Shiffman and Ferguson, 2008, *Addiction*, 103, 557-563.

- Your doctor may advise against pre-quit use of the patch if you have severe heart disease or are pregnant or breastfeeding.

- It's unlikely, but if you have symptoms of too much nicotine—nausea, dizziness, fast or irregular heartbeat—that are not relieved by smoking fewer cigarettes, remove the patch. If you don't feel better soon, call your doctor.

Nicotine Gum and Lozenge

Nicotine gum and lozenges are available without a prescription, in many flavors, and in *what are called* 2 and 4 milligram strengths. However, you only absorb half the nicotine from each piece. The "4 mg" lozenge, for example, gives you just 2 mg of nicotine.

Should I use gum or lozenges?

I usually recommend lozenges because they are easier to use correctly than nicotine gum. Whichever you choose, consider using the nicotine patch along with it.

Should I use the 2 or 4 mg strength?

Use the 4 mg gum or lozenge if you smoked 11 or more cigarettes a day, the 2 mg strength if you smoked fewer. This advice is different (and I think better) than the instructions on the product packages.

How should I use gum or lozenges?

Starting on your quit date, use a piece of gum or lozenge every waking hour. Use extra when needed to relieve cravings and withdrawal symptoms. Use less if you have nausea, dizziness, fast or irregular heartbeat. Do not eat or drink anything other than water for 15 minutes before or while using the gum or lozenge—food and drink interfere with nicotine absorption.

Nicotine lozenge. Let a lozenge dissolve slowly in your mouth. You may notice a warm or tingling sensation in your mouth. Don't chew or swallow the lozenge. Once in a while move it from one side of your mouth to the other.

Nicotine gum. Slowly chew the gum until you notice a peppery taste or a slight tingling in your mouth (after about 15 chews). Then let the gum sit between your cheek and gum. After about a minute, when the taste or tingle is almost gone, chew a few times until the taste returns. Then again place the piece between your cheek and gum. Use each piece this way for about 30 minutes.

What are the side effects?

If you use the gum or lozenges too often, or chew the gum quickly, you may experience indigestion, nausea, hiccups, coughing, or headache.

How long should I use gum or lozenges?

Use frequently for six weeks. Then, after you have gone 14 days in a row without strong cravings or withdrawal symptoms, begin to slowly taper off.

Don't worry if you continue to use some gum or lozenges for many months. The important thing is to stay smokefree. Even after you stop regular use, carry some in case you need it.

www.commitlozenge.com
www.nicorette.com

NICOTINE NASAL SPRAY

Nicotrol® nasal spray is available by prescription. It gets nicotine to the brain faster than other nicotine medicines. This means fast relief from cravings. The spray may be for you if you're a heavy smoker who has tried other medicines without getting enough relief from cravings.

What are the side effects?

When using the nasal spray, you'll probably have a peppery feeling in your nose and throat, cough or sneeze, and have a runny nose. These symptoms usually last several days or weeks, but get better over time. You should not use the spray if you have sinus or breathing problems.

How should I use the spray?

Start the nasal spray on your quit date. Blow your nose if it is not clear. Tilt your head back slightly and spray once into each nostril, spraying to the side of each nostril rather than straight up. Don't sniff, inhale, or swallow while spraying. Just keep a tissue nearby to use if you have a runny nose.

Use the spray once each waking hour. Use more if needed to control cravings, but not more than five times in an hour. Use less if you have nausea, dizziness, rapid or irregular heartbeat. Continue on the spray for at least three months. Then, when you have gone 14 days without strong cravings or withdrawal symptoms, gradually decrease use over three months. Stop when you are comfortable without it.

www.nicotrol.com

The prescription Nicotrol® inhaler looks like a fat cigarette. You load it with nicotine cartridges that also have a bit of menthol.

You will need to puff very frequently on the inhaler—it takes ten puffs to get the nicotine in one drag on most cigarettes. The frequent puffing makes the inhaler a good choice if you have a strong hand-to-mouth habit. However, to get enough nicotine, most people benefit from using the patch in addition to the inhaler.

How should I use the inhaler?

Start using the inhaler on your quit date. The nicotine is absorbed through your mouth and throat so you don't need to inhale deeply. Just take a lot of shallow puffs.

Each cartridge lasts for about 20 minutes of frequent puffing. Use 6 to 16 inhaler cartridges a day for the first three months, and gradually use less over three more months.

Do not eat or drink anything other than water for 15 minutes before or while using the inhaler—food and drink interfere with nicotine absorption. The inhaler doesn't work well if it's cold so if you're outside on a cold day (< 40° F), store the inhaler in an inside pocket.

What are the side effects?

You may notice mild mouth and throat irritation, cough, and a runny nose—these will get better over time.

www.nicotrol.com

Prescription Chantix® reduces nicotine craving and withdrawal symptoms. It partially blocks nicotine's effects and increases the brain's pleasure chemical, dopamine. Chantix has proven very effective in helping people quit smoking, tripling the chance of success.

Is it safe?

Six million people in the U.S. have taken Chantix, the vast majority without serious problems. But a small percentage of Chantix users—several hundred people—have had serious problems that *might* have been caused by Chantix.

These problems include erratic behavior, agitation, depression, suicidal thoughts, and suicide attempts. Some Chantix users have been injured or killed in falls and accidents after experiencing confusion, dizziness, loss of consciousness, visual disturbances, or muscle spasms.

While it is unlikely that you will experience any of these problems, if you or your family suspects a problem or notices any behavior not typical for you, stop taking Chantix and call your doctor.

How should I use Chantix?

Begin Chantix one week before your quit date. Take Chantix after eating and with a full glass of water. Don't take Chantix close to your bedtime. Use caution driving or operating machinery until you know how Chantix affects you.

Week 1. Take a white 0.5 mg tablet once a day for the first 3 days, then twice a day (morning and evening) for days 4–7.

Week 2–12. Starting on day 8, your quit date, take a blue 1.0 mg tablet twice a day, one in the morning and one in the evening.

Week 13–26. If Chantix helped you, staying on it 12 more weeks will increase your chance of continued success.

What are the side effects?

Upset stomach and sleep problems are each reported by a third to half of Chantix users.

Upset stomach. Nausea is most common, with other users reporting gas or constipation.

Sleep problems. Trouble sleeping or vivid and unusual dreams are common.

These symptoms usually get better over time. Call your doctor if side effects are very bothersome or persistent. You may be told to cut back to one tablet a day. The one-tablet dose doubles your chance of success.

Can I use nicotine products with Chantix?

Do not combine the nicotine patch with Chantix—one study found this caused a lot of nausea and other side effects. However, if you still crave cigarettes while using Chantix, ask your doctor about adding some 2 mg nicotine lozenges or gum. Most people find this helps without increasing side effects.

www.chantix.com

Prescription Zyban® reduces the desire to smoke and lessens withdrawal symptoms. A low-cost generic form of Zyban, bupropion ER, is also available. It's not clear how Zyban works, but like smoking it mildly improves one's mood.

Zyban contains the same medicine as the antidepressant Wellbutrin®, but you don't have to have problems with depression for Zyban to help you quit smoking.

How should I use Zyban?

Start Zyban one to two weeks before your quit date, and continue taking it for seven to twelve weeks. If Zyban helps you and your doctor approves, you can stay on it for up to six months.

Two-tablet dose. Doctors usually say to take a 150 mg tablet each morning for the first three days, and from then on to add a second daily tablet in the early evening.

One-tablet dose. Two studies found that people who take just one 150 mg tablet a day are about as successful as those taking two tablets. The one-tablet option has less risk of side effects and costs less. Generic Zyban is available at Wal-Mart for about $30 for a two month supply. Talk with your doctor about the one-tablet option.

What are the side effects?

About a third of users have trouble sleeping and one in ten experiences a dry mouth. These problems often get better over a few weeks. If you have trouble sleeping, be sure you are not taking Zyban close to your bedtime.

There is also a positive side effect of using Zyban. It delays about half the weight gain that can occur when you quit smoking. I say *delays* because when you stop taking Zyban you may put on a bit of weight.

Precautions

Check with your doctor before using Zyban if you are pregnant or breastfeeding. There is a slight risk of seizure in some people taking Zyban. Avoid Zyban if you have had:

- Seizure disorder.

- Eating disorder (bulimia, anorexia nervosa).

- Severe head injury or brain tumor.

- Alcohol or sedative withdrawal recently.

- Wellbutrin (bupropion) use recently.

- MAO inhibitor use in the past 2 weeks (Azilect, Eldepryl, Marplan, Nardil, Parnate).

Zyban plus nicotine patches

Zyban doubles your chance of success, compared to not using stop-smoking medicine. Your chance of success increases 2.5 times when you use both Zyban and the nicotine patch. In some people, taking the two medicines together increases blood pressure so have your blood pressure checked.

LET FAMILY AND FRIENDS HELP

Many people pride themselves on being self-reliant, independent, and strong-willed. They try to quit smoking by toughing it out alone, without the support of others. Some people do not even tell others that they are trying to quit. That is not quitting smart.

You are most likely to succeed when you ask for support. You will want a support person at home, at work, and in social situations. Tell these people that you plan to quit and discuss how they can help. You might ask them to:

- Read this guide so they understand your quitting program.

- Go with you on smoke-free activities (a walk, a movie).

- Help talk you through urges.

- Praise you for not smoking.

- Give you rewards (hugs, cards, flowers).

- Not remind you of past difficulties in quitting.

- Be tolerant of your withdrawal symptoms (irritability, nervousness).

- Not nag or attempt to police you.

- Remind you that withdrawal symptoms will pass.

- Point out positive changes (you look healthier, breathe easier).

- Express confidence in your ability to remain a nonsmoker.

- Realize that you can use special support for a full year.

Review this list with your support people so you can plan the best support strategy. Do not be shy about doing this. Your family and friends want you alive and well, and will be pleased when you request their help.

A few weeks after your quit date, let your family and friends know how much you appreciate their support by sending each person a thank you note or a small gift.

List your support people

At home: _____

At work: _____

A friend: _____

Avoid Smoking Triggers

Before you quit, smoke proof your home, car, and workplace. After quitting, avoid things that serve as triggers for smoking.

Destroy your cigarettes. Just before your quit date, destroy all your cigarettes. The sight and smell of cigarettes will only tempt you. Be sure you search out every last cigarette and cigarette butt and destroy them completely! Also, remove ash trays and lighters.

Avoid smokers. For your first few weeks as a nonsmoker, avoid being around people who are smoking. Do not schedule lunch dates or social outings with smokers during this risky time. Ask close friends and relatives not to smoke around you.

For the long term, make a point of getting to know your nonsmoking friends better. By spending more time with these friends, you will be more likely to remain smokefree.

Avoid smoky places. Smoky places serve as triggers for smoking. Try to avoid smoking-allowed bars, restaurants, bowling alleys, coffee-break areas, and parties where people may be smoking. Even places in your own home or office that you associate with cigarettes, such as your favorite "smoking chair," should be avoided for a time.

George's story. George quit smoking but suffered much longer than most people. Several weeks after quitting, he was still irritable and anxious, and had lots of urges for a cigarette. With each urge, he debated: "Should I smoke or not? Maybe I could have just one."

Then something happened. His best buddy, a smoker, was diagnosed with lung cancer. This hit George very hard. Cigarettes were killing his best friend. George decided—*really decided*—that he would never smoke again, that he was a nonsmoker no matter what! Incredibly, the withdrawal symptoms disappeared. He suffered no more irritability, no more "nerves," and he had few urges to smoke.

Stop the debate. Once George decided that he would never smoke again, the internal debate ended. It was this constant debate, the back and forth thoughts about whether or not to have a cigarette, that caused his long suffering.

Once you really decide you are a nonsmoker, urges are not relevant. You no longer have to think about cigarettes all the time, and your mind can go on to more pleasant things.

If you have not yet made a firm decision to quit for good, think it through one last time. It may not be an easy decision. If despite mixed feelings, you decide that you want most to quit, make your decision and do not debate it further. When you make a firm decision to quit, you will be surprised at how easy quitting can be.

SELECT YOUR QUIT DATE

If you have not already done so, now is the time to select your quit date. This will be your first day of freedom from cigarettes. Your quit date should be one to three weeks in the future to allow time to:

- Arrange for the support of family and friends.

- Reduce your nicotine intake by switching to cigarette brands that deliver less nicotine.

- Talk to your doctor about medications to help you quit. You begin some of the medicines 1–2 weeks before your quit date so you'll need to plan ahead.

- Prepare urge-control methods by studying the *Quitting* chapter of this guide.

- Destroy all your cigarettes, and remove ashtrays (just before your quit date).

If possible, select a quit date that will not be stressful, perhaps a Saturday or a vacation day. Complete the Stop Tobacco Contract on the next page.

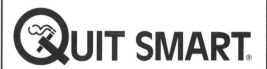

Stop Tobacco Contract

I will stop all tobacco use on

5.16.13

(date)

and do all I can to stay free of tobacco

Your signature

5.2.13

Date

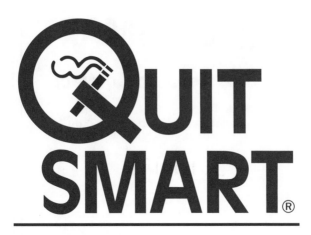

CHAPTER 2
Quitting

Hats off to you for getting this far, and for devoting the time and energy to plan ahead for successful quitting.

You are now ready to quit. You have a lot of tools to help you succeed. On your quit date you will start listening to your hypnosis CD and start using your fake cigarette. You may also begin using the nicotine gum, lozenge, nasal spray, or inhaler, and begin or continue to use the patch. If you are taking Zyban or Chantix tablets, you will continue to do so.

In this chapter, you will learn to keep withdrawal symptoms in perspective and to *actively do things to cope*. You will learn to relax, to use coping methods that help control cigarette urges, and to use your thoughts to make nonsmoking easier.

You will see why, as a nonsmoker, you may need less coffee, tea, and cola. However, you will not be asked to give up caffeine entirely.

Keep using the methods you have already learned: call on your family and friends for support, avoid people who smoke and places where smoking occurs, and refer often to your list of reasons for quitting.

The quitting phase lasts about a week. Then your task turns to remaining a nonsmoker. Look ahead at Chapter 3, *Remaining a Nonsmoker*, so you will be prepared for this challenge.

LEARN TO RELAX

Many people suffer from tension and tension-related symptoms such as upset stomach, headaches, difficulty sleeping, and tiredness. Withdrawal from cigarettes may produce a temporary increase in tension. By practicing the relaxation methods discussed below, you will learn to relax while keeping your mind clear and sharp.

Take a breather Much of the relaxation you get from smoking a cigarette is due to pausing and taking several slow deep breaths. Try taking a breather.

- Take a slow breath, drawing the air deep into your lungs.

- Hold the breath a few seconds.

- Exhale slowly as you relax and say to yourself *calm* or *relax*.

- Repeat this sequence several times.

Take a breather at least twenty times a day. Use daily events to remind you. For example, take a breather when you hang up the phone, during television ads, when you feel annoyed, and whenever you can use a break. Also, take a breather if you have an urge for a cigarette.

Add physical activity For example, take a daily walk or ride a bike. Move everyday, but don't overdo it—starting a difficult exercise program can add stress rather than reduce it.

Solve sleep problems. If you have trouble sleeping, be sure you are not drinking something with caffeine (coffee, tea, or cola) within six hours of bedtime. Also, avoid naps.

Your sleep should improve a week or two after quitting. As a nonsmoker, you may need less sleep than you did as a smoker. For example, you might be able to stay up 15 minutes later before going to bed.

If you are wearing a nicotine patch at night and have difficulty falling asleep or have overly vivid dreams, this could be a side-effect of the patch. Try removing the patch an hour before bedtime. Zyban and Chantix can also disrupt sleep—call your doctor if this is a problem.

Use physical methods to relax. Hot baths, massage, stretching exercises, a hot-water bottle, and relaxing music are all calming. Each of these can be used as often as you wish and require no outside help (even massage can be self-massage).

Take vitamins. Stress can rob you of vitamins and minerals. If your doctor does not object, take a multivitamin.

Remember, you will soon feel better. Within three months of breaking free from cigarettes, most exsmokers report feeling more relaxed and happy than they felt while smoking.

Hypnosis is simply relaxation with focused attention. It is a way to use the full power of your mind to become a nonsmoker. There is no magic; you remain in control.

Start using the *QuitSmart Hypnosis CD* on your quit date. The deep voice of Robert Conroy will help you relax and enjoy life as a nonsmoker. If you do not have this CD, see the order form on the last page of this guide.

Track One of the CD, *Quitting*, eases you through your first few weeks of freedom from cigarettes. The suggestions on the CD help you relax and enjoy healthy pleasures, as you avoid unwanted weight gain or other negative effects.

Track Two, *Remaining a Nonsmoker*, helps to instill the feelings of inner calm and strength that are most helpful in staying free of cigarettes for a lifetime.

What is hypnosis?

Hypnosis is relaxation with focused attention. You have probably been in a hypnotic state while watching a good movie or listening to music. Whenever you relax and become so focused on one thing that you are not easily distracted, you are using the powerful state of mind called hypnosis.

How should I use the hypnosis CD?

Start using the CD on your quit date. Pick a time and place where you will not be disturbed for at least 15 minutes. Turn the lights down, get comfortable in a chair, sofa, or bed that supports all parts of your body. Start the player and relax.

How often should I listen to the CD?

The more times you listen to the CD, the better. Start listening to Track One, *Quitting*, on your quit date. Listen at least twice daily during your first week off cigarettes. The next week, listen to Track One once daily, and listen to Track Two, *Remaining a Nonsmoker*, once a day. After that, listen to Track One or Two as often as you want or need to, listening most often to the track you find more relaxing and helpful.

What if I don't have time to listen?

Do yourself a favor—make time! It only takes 15 minutes. Even if you have to wake up 15 minutes earlier in the morning to listen to the CD, you'll feel better and have more energy than if you slept in.

How will I know if I was in a hypnotic state?

You will simply feel relaxed, your hands may feel heavy and warm, or they may tingle. In any case, you do not need to be in a deep hypnotic state to benefit from the CD.

Should I concentrate hard and try to remember everything on the CD?

No. Just relax and listen to the voice on the CD without concentrating on every word. Listen to the voice but do not worry about the words too much.

What if I get stuck in hypnosis?

You cannot get stuck in the hypnotic state. The hypnotic state is between sleep and wakefulness; you pass through this state when you fall asleep and again when you wake up. If you are tired when you listen to the CD, you could fall asleep. You would wake up as you normally do—when you are rested, or when there is a noise or someone calls your name.

Can I use the CD to help me fall asleep?

Yes, but the suggestions on the CD are most helpful if you are in the hypnotic state between sleep and wakefulness. It is best to listen to the CD and then allow yourself to go to sleep. The instructions at the end of Track Two may help—they tell you to return to your normal waking state, unless you have decided to use the CD to fall asleep.

Is it alright to use the CD while driving?

No. Since hypnosis can make you sleepy, DO NOT LISTEN WHILE DRIVING OR USING MACHINES.

Are there added benefits from the CD?

It will help you relax more quickly and completely. This can reduce stress symptoms such as headaches, upset stomach, irritability, and sleep problems.

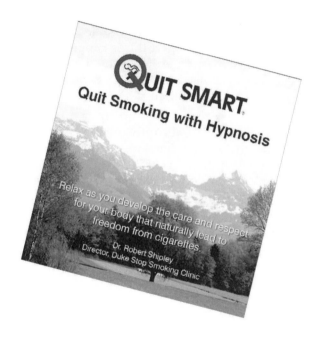

REDUCE CAFFEINE?

Many smokers consume a lot of caffeine. Caffeine is a stimulant found in coffee, tea, soft drinks, energy drinks, chocolate, and some medicines. Smokers clear caffeine from their bodies faster than do nonsmokers. That is one reason many smokers drink so much coffee and cola.

Over several weeks after you stop smoking, caffeine will stay in your body longer and longer. This gradually could make you feel nervous and jittery. If you suspect this is happening, try reducing your caffeine intake by a third. For example, if you used to drink six cups of coffee a day, cut back to four cups.

Do not cut back too much—caffeine is addictive. If you abruptly swear off most caffeine, you could suffer withdrawal symptoms such as headaches, irritability, and sleepiness. You do not need these symptoms when you are quitting smoking.

Caffeine Content

Coffee	Average Mg
Starbucks Tall (12 oz)	260
McDonalds Large (16 oz)	145
Coffee, brewed (8 oz)	110
Espresso (2 oz)	100
Coffee, instant (8 oz)	80
Starbucks Cappuccino (12 oz)	75

Tea	
Black tea (8 oz)	50
Green tea (8 oz)	20

Soft Drinks, 12 oz	
Pepsi Max, diet	69
Mountain Dew (regular, diet)	55
Pepsi One	54
Mello Yello	53
Coke, diet	46
Dr. Pepper (regular, diet)	41
Sunkist Orange	41
Pepsi-Cola (regular, diet)	38
Coca-Cola (Classic, Zero)	35

www.energyfiend.com

New exsmokers are like newcomers to a nudist resort—they don't know what to do with their hands. The QuitSmart cigarette substitute gives you something to do with your hands and mouth. It looks and feels like a real cigarette. The fake cigarette also reminds you to take deep, relaxing breaths—just like you did when you smoked. (To order, see page 94)

You smoked primarily to get a hit of nicotine to your brain. The look and feel of a cigarette became pleasurable because you associated the cigarette with this hit of nicotine. The fake cigarette will help you break this association. Since it has no nicotine, use of the substitute gradually lessens the pleasure associated with the look and feel of a cigarette.

Begin using the cigarette substitute on your quit date. Adjust the air flow to your liking by sliding the filter in or out. Take deep draws of fresh air, and enjoy relaxing. Use the carrying case to keep the substitute clean and handy.

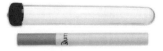

Carry the cigarette substitute in your pocket or purse and use it whenever you are tempted to smoke. Gradually, the power of these situations to tempt you will decrease. When the cigarette substitute no longer gives you pleasure, stop regular use. However, continue to carry it to help with rare urges for a cigarette.

The mind has the power to create feelings out of thin air. For example, you may be able to create hunger by thinking about a juicy steak, or sleepiness by imagining a yawn coming on.

This power of the mind can be used in three ways to help you stay free from cigarettes. You can use your thoughts to create a nonsmoking self-image, to control cigarette urges by focusing on something else, and to keep life's hassles in perspective.

Create a nonsmoking self-image. A person's self-image has a powerful effect on behavior. When you think of yourself as a nonsmoker, you will behave as a nonsmoker. You will, for example, sit in the nonsmoking section of restaurants. If you feel bored or anxious, you will not interpret those feelings as an urge for a cigarette because nonsmokers do not have such urges.

The effect of self-image on behavior is well known in sports. Greg Louganis became a world champion diver, in part, by thinking of himself as a great diver and by imagining himself performing each dive perfectly. I sometimes improve my tennis play by imagining that I'm Roger Federer. As "Roger," I'm a stronger, more confident tennis player.

You are what you believe. Believing you are a permanent nonsmoker will naturally lead to that outcome. Do not make the mistake of seeing yourself as a smoker who is not smoking. You would feel deprived and depressed.

If you have trouble seeing yourself as a nonsmoker, do what Alcoholics Anonymous suggests to its members, "Fake it till you make it." Pretend you're a calm, comfortable nonsmoker until that becomes true for you.

Focus on pleasant thoughts. Most urges for a cigarette can be controlled by thinking about something else. Focusing on an urge is like focusing on an itchy nose—it will drive you crazy. Instead, turn your thoughts to something pleasant, like a walk on the beach.

Keep hassles in perspective. You may know people who get very upset with the least little mishap, and other people who handle a crisis calmly. The ability to roll with the punches will be important during your first few weeks without cigarettes.

The key to maintaining perspective is to realize that the way you think about a situation determines your feelings about it. For example, when caught in a traffic jam, you can make yourself very angry by thinking, "I'll never be on time; this is awful," or relatively calm by thinking, "This is a chance to take a breather and enjoy the radio."

Your thoughts can make quitting smoking either difficult or relatively easy. Quitting will be difficult if you tell yourself that withdrawal symptoms are terrible. Instead, tell yourself that you accept some discomfort, and that you are adding freedom and self-control to your life. With positive thinking, quitting can be surprisingly easy and fulfilling.

Shakespeare wrote, "There is nothing either good or bad, but thinking makes it so." (*Hamlet*, Act II, Scene 2) Using your thoughts wisely will help you stay calm and avoid making "mountains out of molehills."

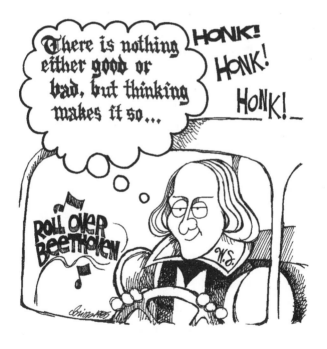

WITHDRAWL SYMPTOMS

At first the challenge of breaking free of cigarettes is getting through physical withdrawal. Your body is used to getting nicotine in hundreds of daily puffs. The use of brand switching and medication will reduce any discomfort, but you may briefly experience some of the following symptoms:

- Frustration, irritability, anger

- Sadness, depression

- Difficulty sleeping

- Anxiety

- Restlessness

- Difficulty concentrating

- Cravings for tobacco

- Hunger

- Fatigue

- Dizziness

- Tingling in arms and legs

- Constipation

- Sweating

- Coughing

Each person has different symptoms. For example, some people feel tense, while others feel drowsy. Many people have little discomfort. Any symptoms you have are temporary and are a sign that your body is healing itself.

Withdrawal symptoms are temporary. They peak during the first three to six days, and mostly disappear within two to four weeks. Soon after that, you will be healthier and calmer than you were as a smoker.

Urges are short-lived. It may seem that an urge lasts forever, but actually an urge peaks and subsides within three to five minutes. If you interrupt an urge with a coping method (deep breaths, pleasant thoughts), you will conquer it even sooner.

Withdrawal symptoms are a sign that your body is healing itself.

- Tingling in your arms and legs results from better blood flow.

- Feeling dizzy or lightheaded occurs as your brain gets more oxygen than it is used to.

- Coughing may increase for a few days as your lung's hair-like cilia, no longer paralyzed by tobacco smoke, work overtime to remove tar from your lungs.

- Increased sweating may occur as chemicals from tobacco smoke are flushed out of your body through the skin's pores.

Use coping methods. Take deep relaxing breaths, use your fake cigarette, and listen to the hypnosis CD. If constipation is a problem, drink plenty of water and add more fiber to your diet.

Consider increasing nicotine medication. If you are using a nicotine-replacement medicine and still have bothersome withdrawal symptoms, consider increasing your nicotine dose—use more of your current medicine or add a second nicotine medicine.

Focus on positive changes. Look for the first signs of physical and mental improvement. After a few days to a week off cigarettes:

- Oxygen level in your blood increases to normal, and carbon monoxide level decreases to normal—you can walk farther without feeling winded.

- Blood flow improves—your hands and feet are warmer, and your skin is rosier, healthier.

- Your heart is healthier—blood pressure and heart rate come down to a healthier level. Your risk of a heart attack decreases.

- Your sinuses clear.

- Your teeth and fingers are cleaner.

- Your senses of smell and taste improve.

- You have a sense of rebirth and pride in your success.

REDUCED DISEASE RISK

Your risk of suffering serious disease drops over the years that you remain free of cigarettes.

One to two years

- Excess risk of heart attack is 40–50% less than for a continuing smoker.

Five to ten years

- Stroke risk is reduced to near that of people who never smoked.

Ten to fifteen years

- Heart attack risk is similar to people who never smoked.

- Lung cancer risk drops to as little as half that of continuing smokers.

- Risk of other cancers (mouth, throat, kidney, etc.) is greatly reduced.

- Overall risk of premature death returns to nearly that of people who never smoked.

The smoking habit may be strong, but it is also dumb—you can outsmart it! Small changes in your habits can reduce your urges to smoke. Try the following:

- **Leave the table after a meal.** Brush your teeth or take a walk. This will help break the association between finishing a meal and having a cigarette.

- **Change habits associated with smoking.** If you smoked while talking on the phone, talk in a different room, hold the phone in the other hand, or sit in a different chair. If you usually smoked while sitting in your favorite chair, avoid that chair for a while.

- **Change work breaks.** For many smokers, a cigarette and a break go together. So, change your break routine—go to a different location (smokefree), and take deep relaxing breaths or use oral substitutes.

- **Keep busy.** Take up a hobby, go to the movies, go for a walk, work around the house, call or visit friends, write letters, send email, or read a book.

- **Increase physical activity.** Walk daily or play a sport. The next time you need a pick-me-up, try some jumping jacks or a walk in the fresh air.

- **Keep your hands and mouth busy.** Use your fake cigarette. You may also want to try sugarless mints or gum, toothpicks, cinnamon sticks, carrot and celery sticks, crushed ice and water.

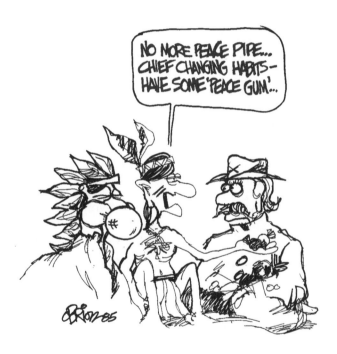

Drink plenty of fluids. Drink lots of water and other beverages to help flush the cigarette poisons from your body.

Avoid swings in blood sugar. Eat regular meals with lots of fruit, vegetables, and protein. Avoid foods that contain a lot of sugar.

Relax. Take a breather many times a day and whenever you have an urge to smoke.

Remind yourself that urges will pass. An urge passes within three to five minutes—you can wait it out.

Think about what you will buy. Plan how you will spend the money no longer wasted on cigarettes and medical bills.

Ask friends and relatives for help. Tell them you are quitting and how they can help.

Praise yourself. Think often of your pride at resisting cigarettes. Mentally pat yourself on the back each time you outsmart an urge.

Focus on positive changes. When you first quit smoking, it's tempting to focus on any discomfort. Intead, focus on positive changes. For example, if your sense of smell has improved or you are breathing easier, focus your thoughts on these improvements.

Express your frustrations. Gently stick up for your rights, or pound a pillow, or take a walk. Do something with your frustrations; do not let them serve as an excuse for a cigarette.

Phone for help. Call 1-800-QUIT-NOW (1-800-784-8669) for free advice and support. If you are using stop-smoking medicine, call the support numbers provided with these products.

Visit stop-smoking websites.

www.QuitSmart.com

www.smokefree.gov

www.cdc.gov/tobacco

www.quitnet.com

Feel proud. When you see someone having a cigarette, feel proud that you no longer have such a harmful addiction. Let yourself feel a bit superior and smug.

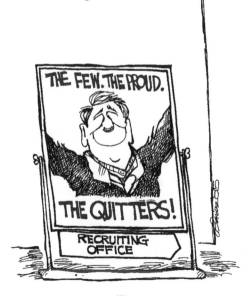

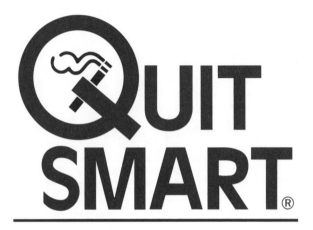

CHAPTER 3
Remaining a Nonsmoker

Congratulations! You are over the worst. From here on, urges become less frequent. Now your task turns to staying a nonsmoker over the long haul. This chapter will prepare you to overcome situations that often lead new exsmokers to fall off the wagon.

Relapse is most common during periods of negative emotions (anger, frustration, anxiety, or depression). To keep your mood on an even keel, you will learn to increase the positives in your life and decrease the negatives. Continued use of your relaxation skills (taking a breather, daily walks) and of stop-smoking medication will also help control negative emotions.

Relapse occurs for some people when others pressure them to have *just one*. You will learn firm responses to such smoking come-ons. Likewise, you may be tempted by your own thoughts ("I need a cigarette to handle this crisis"), and firm responses are needed here too. You will learn the folly of thinking you can smoke just one cigarette.

Finally, weight gain, which may or may not be due to quitting smoking, often serves as an excuse for relapse. Instead, you will learn to control your weight by eating sensibly and by using coping methods similar to those you used to overcome smoking.

Now that you have given up the pleasure of smoking, it is important to increase other pleasures in your daily life. Bing Crosby sang:

You've got to Accentuate The Positive
Eliminate The Negative
Latch on to The Affirmative
Don't mess around with Mister Inbetween.

LYRICS BY JOHNNY MERCER

If you have too many negatives in your day, and not enough positives, you can get frustrated and depressed. It can be tempting to smoke in order to feel better.

Instead, add some positives: appreciate the little things in life such as a beautiful sunset, do something each day that gives you pleasure, buy gifts for yourself, and think pleasant thoughts. Also, be on the lookout for negatives you can eliminate.

Many new exsmokers fail to act on these ideas because they have trouble being nice to themselves; but so much depends on your taking action—your happiness, the happiness of those around you, and your health.

Get some ideas from the following lists of ways other exsmokers have added positives and eliminated negatives. Then make your own lists of positives you will accentuate, and negatives you will eliminate.

Positives added

- Karen took pleasant walks after dinner.
- Jill treated herself to a bubble bath.
- Jack started getting a massage each week.
- Ron paused for slow deep breaths.
- Sue bought flowers every week.
- Rod bought several compact discs.
- Bert focused on life's little pleasures.

Little Things

Most of us miss out on life's big prizes
The Pulitzer, The Nobel, Oscars, Tonys, Emmys
But we're all eligible for life's small pleasures
A pat on the back
A kiss behind the ear
A four-pound bass, A full moon
An empty parking space
A crackling fire, A great meal, A glorious sunset
Hot soup
Cold beer
Don't fret about copping life's grand awards
Enjoy its tiny delights
There are plenty for all of us

—*Anonymous*

Positives I Will Accentuate

_____

_____

_____

_____

_____

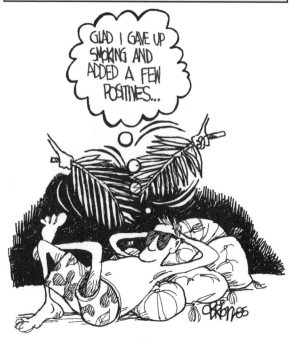

Negatives eliminated

- Mary resigned from a committee that she disliked.

- Elaine got rid of phone calls during the family dinner by unplugging the phone.

- Sam decided to stop feeling guilty for wanting some time to himself.

- Steve traded his least favorite chore— loading the dishwasher—for walking the dog, a pleasant way of increasing exercise.

- Jackie decided to take some time off work to do things she enjoys.

Negatives I Will Eliminate
_____
_____
_____
_____
_____
_____

REBUFF SMOKING COME-ONS

Most people will try to help you stay free of cigarettes, but a few may try to tempt you to smoke. This can happen because your success threatens them or because they are impatient with your irritability or other withdrawal symptoms. It pays to prepare yourself to stand up for your decision to remain a nonsmoker.

Smoking Come-on	Possible Response
Have a cigarette, just one won't hurt.	No, it's stupid to tempt fate. I'm glad to be a nonsmoker.
You're so irritable; have a cigarette.	I may be irritable, but I'm not crazy Please don't offer me a cigarette.
We're having such a good time; join me in a cigarette.	I don't smoke anymore. Why don't you join me for a walk?
Congratulations on a good job. You deserve a cigarette.	I don't smoke, but I'll have some tea.
Have a cigarette; you're going to die sooner or later anyway.	No thanks, I'd prefer later.

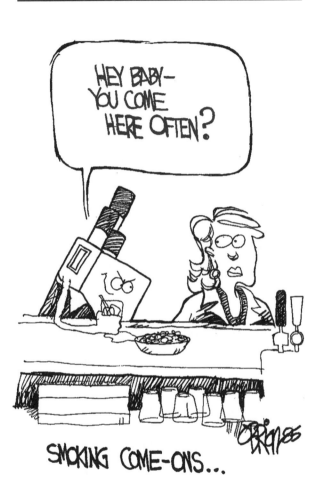

SMOKING COME-ONS...

As you read the smoking come-ons, you may have realized that you have used some of these against yourself. Perhaps you told yourself "have just one" or "have a cigarette to calm down" or "you deserve a cigarette."

When this happens, be just as forceful with yourself as you will be if somebody else goes against your decision to be free of cigarettes. Look back over the come-ons on page 74 and put a check mark by any that you have used against yourself.

Listed below are other common self come-ons and possible responses.

Self Come-on	Possible Response
Nostalgia: Smoking was so great with coffee.	Maybe, but there were also times cigarettes tasted bad.
Crisis: I can't handle this without a cigarette.	No, a cigarette only makes me feel more defeated. I'll take a few deep breaths and handle this.
Anger: I'll show that so-and-so; I'll smoke a cigarette.	I'll stick up for myself and stick by my decision to be a nonsmoker.
Defeatism: Since I'm a jerk anyway, I may as well smoke.	Nobody's perfect, but I'm proud that I quit smoking.

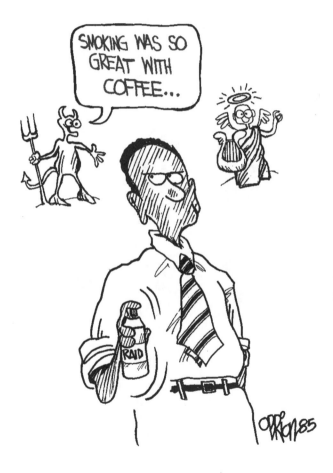

Did you know that among exsmokers who have *just one* cigarette, nine out of ten soon return to regular smoking? After two cigarettes, the odds are even worse. Some exsmokers think they can beat the odds—but why try? Other exsmokers want to smoke just one to prove how strong they are. However, it shows more strength to resist temptation.

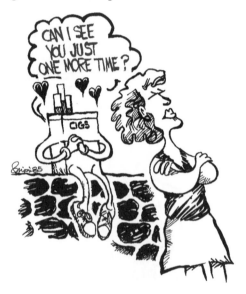

Exsmokers who have one cigarette feel guilty and discouraged. They think of themselves as smokers. Believing that the battle is already lost, they go back to regular smoking—"I already blew it, so I might as well smoke another."

You have made a wise decision to quit smoking and have invested lots of time and energy to become a nonsmoker. It makes sense to protect your investment by never allowing yourself *just one*.

Dwight Eisenhower quit smoking in 1949 after he had a (probable) heart attack. It wasn't easy to quit—he had been a four-pack-a-day smoker. At a press conference, President Eisenhower said, "I don't know whether I will start smoking but I will never stop again."

By never having a cigarette you will never again have to quit smoking. Underscore your determination to stay completely free of tobacco by signing the contract below.

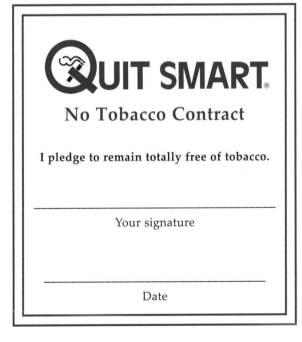

QUIT SMART®

No Tobacco Contract

I pledge to remain totally free of tobacco.

_____

Your signature

_____

Date

Weight gain is a prime reason some people give for going back to smoking. Four out of five people who quit smoking gain some weight.

Without the stimulation of nicotine, your body uses fewer calories. Despite needing fewer calories, you may eat more because food tastes better, and because eating serves as an oral substitute for smoking.

Accept some weight gain. Try to accept a few added pounds as a trade off for feeling better and living longer. If you gain more than five or ten pounds, devise a weight control strategy. However, if you try to lose weight quickly or too soon after quitting smoking, you are likely to return to smoking.

Eat sensibly. To control your weight, avoid starvation diets, fad diets, and diet pills. Eat regular meals with lots of fresh fruit and vegetables, and plenty of lean protein (fish, poultry, beans). Allow yourself some snacks so you don't feel deprived. Avoid sugar or corn syrup (soft drinks) and refined carbohydrates (white rice, pasta, potatoes). Whole grains are fine (oatmeal, brown rice, whole-wheat bread).

Apply your new skills. Many of the methods that helped you stay off cigarettes can also help control your weight.

- **Relax**. Take a breather to relax and control the urge to overeat.

- **Stay active**. A daily walk reduces stress, lessens hunger, and burns calories.

- **Use medication**. Stop-smoking medicines, especially Zyban, may reduce weight gain.

- **Avoid temptation**. Do not keep fattening foods in the house.

- **See yourself as a healthy eater**. Remember *thinking makes it so*. Think of yourself as a person who is very selective about what you eat, a picky eater who always leaves some food on your plate.

- **Control the enemy within.** Look back at *Control the Enemy Within* (page 76) and plan how you will respond to similar thoughts that tempt you to go off your sensible-eating plan.

- **Use rewards**. When you eat sensibly, reward yourself. Avoid depression and anger by increasing the positives in your life.

- **Listen to your hypnosis CD**. Track One includes weight control suggestions.

Stay smokefree. If you gain weight, don't be tempted to go back to smoking. Most people who go back to cigarettes do not lose much weight. Accept some weight gain as a normal part of gaining your freedom from cigarettes. For a large weight gain, tackle it only after you are confident that you'll remain a nonsmoker.

Often smokers avoid learning the harmful effects of cigarettes because these effects are so frightening. However, now that you are free of cigarettes, knowing the dangers of smoking will strengthen your resolve to remain a nonsmoker.

Health problems of smokers

- Heart disease
- Cancers of the lung, mouth, larynx, colon, esophagus, bladder, kidney, pancreas, breast, liver, stomach, and sex organs
- Emphysema and bronchitis
- Stroke
- Bone loss (osteoporosis) and increased risk of hip fracture
- Facial wrinkles (due to poor blood flow to the skin, and the drying effects of smoke)
- Headaches
- Mental decline and poor memory
- Major depression
- Cataracts
- Low sex drive, impotence, and decreased fertility
- Premature gray hair and balding
- Early and uncomfortable menopause
- High blood pressure

- Hearing loss (smoke damages the hair-like cells involved in hearing)

- Pregnant smokers may have underweight babies

- Low back pain

- Shortness of breath

- Colds, coughs, and sore throats

Health effects on loved ones

Exposure to second-hand smoke can cause lung cancer in nonsmokers, and increases the chance they will have a stroke or heart disease.

Children living with smokers are twice as likely to become smokers. They also are more likely to suffer from colds, sore throats, asthma, ear infections, bronchitis, and pneumonia.

Some of the 4000 chemicals smokers inhale

Acetaldehyde, acetone, aceturitrile, acrolein, acrylonitrile, ammonia, **arsenic**, benzene, butylamine, carbon monoxide, carbon dioxide, cresols, crotononitrile, dimethylamine, endrin, ethylamine, formaldehyde, furfural hydroquinone, **hydrogen cyanide** (used in the gas chamber), hydrogen sulfide, lead, methacrolein, methyl alcohol, methylamine, nickel compounds, nicotine, nitric oxide, nitrogen dioxide, phenol, **polonium-210** (radioactive), pyridine, tar (burned plant resins)

Benefits of Nonsmoking

Now that you're a nonsmoker, it's important to focus on the benefits you will enjoy. You'll save money, feel better, and much more.

You save money

You no longer waste money on cigarettes, and your medical and insurance costs will be lower. Use the savings to buy things that give you pleasure. Those pleasures will increase your chance of staying a nonsmoker.

Cigarettes. The cost of cigarettes is increasing every year. If cigarettes cost $5.00 a pack, a pack-a-day smoker pays $1,825 each year— that's $36,500 over 20 years! What will you buy with that?

Medical costs. As a nonsmoker, you are less likely to get sick. On average, a 39 year old man who breaks a two-pack-a-day cigarette addiction saves $90,000 over his lifetime in medical bills and in earnings not lost due to illness.

Insurance. Nonsmokers pay less for health, life, car, and home insurance. Smokers pay more for home insurance because they have more house fires. They pay more for car insurance because they have more accidents, possibly because smoking distracts them.

You feel better

You have more energy, you look better, your heart rate is lower, your hands and feet stay warmer due to better circulation, and you are proud of breaking free from cigarettes.

How many benefits are you enjoying?

Below are benefits noted by exsmokers just a few weeks after they quit smoking.

- I feel in control of my life for the first time in fifteen years.

- I like not burning holes in my clothes and furniture.

- I've inspired others to quit.

- I don't believe how calm I am.

- I feel more poised in social situations.

- Now I am a good role model for my kids.

- I feel great!

- I have so much more time.

- It's amazing how much I get done now that I have two hands.

- I enjoy having more money to spend on me.

- No more sinus headaches—it's wonderful.

- My skin is healthy pink instead of ash gray.

- Sour stomach is completely gone.

- Now I can play two sets of tennis without fading from lack of lung power.

- The house is cleaner, and smells fresher.

- My sex drive picked up; I feel ten years younger.

- I eat slower and enjoy my food—don't rush through the meal to get a cigarette.

- I enjoyed the half-time show at a basketball game while the addicts rushed out for a cigarette.

- I feel more attractive—actually, I am more attractive.

- I no longer hide my anger in a cloud of smoke.

- I feel self-confident.

- I'm starting to take better care of myself in other ways.

- I don't have to empty dirty ashtrays ever again.

- I no longer have to feel embarrassed about being a smoker.

- No more tobacco film on my car windows.

- I'm keeping things in better perspective; I now see little hassles as little hassles.

- I no longer have to make excuses about why I'm still smoking.

- Proud that I quit just for me.

- No more angry looks from people whose air is being polluted.

- It's great not to worry about starting an accidental fire.

- I don't have to worry about my smoke hurting others.

- I sleep better and wake up refreshed.
- My heart stopped skipping beats.
- My lover tells me I'm more kissable.
- I climbed the stairs to the third floor and could still talk.
- I feel so strong and competent.
- My husband told me he liked my new perfume—the same one I generally wear but without the smoke smell.
- I love smelling flowers now.
- I'm the envy of the office—they all want to quit now.
- I no longer feel like a social outcast.
- I got my teeth cleaned and they stayed clean.
- I smile more.
- Don't have to worry about always having available a cigarette, lighter, and ashtray.
- I love saying, "I'm a nonsmoker."
- I seem to have more time to enjoy myself.
- I haven't had a cold in months.
- That hacking cough is gone.
- My hair no longer smells like stale smoke.
- I look forward to living a longer life.
- I don't need as much sleep as I used to.

- I feel good about taking better care of my body.

- I no longer worry about a heart attack.

- I enjoy being the resident expert at work on how to quit smoking.

- Nasal passages are clear—I can breathe.

- The pain in my chest is gone.

- No longer cough up black stuff.

- I don't have to hide behind a cigarette anymore.

- I can be close to people without worrying about smoker's breath.

- No longer have to frantically read the signs to see if it's OK to smoke.

- New man I met told me he would never date a smoker.

- Glad I QuitSmart instead of gritting my teeth and suffering.

- I'm so proud.

WHAT'S NEXT?

Continue to use your coping methods. Urges will arise less and less often, but when they do come, they may still be strong. List the coping methods you have found helpful and will continue to use.

```
┌──────────────────────────────────────┐
│                                        │
│          My Coping Methods             │
│                                        │
│  _____  │
│                                        │
│  _____  │
│                                        │
│  _____  │
│                                        │
│  _____  │
│                                        │
│  _____  │
│                                        │
│  _____  │
│                                        │
└──────────────────────────────────────┘
```

Remember to be extra nice to yourself. To prevent or overcome post-quitting blues, be extra nice to yourself—do things you want to do. Use the money you are saving by not smoking to buy things that you will enjoy.

After the challenge of quitting, staying smokefree can seem like a letdown. People around you may be less supportive, thinking you already have it made. So, it is up to you to pamper yourself over the next several months.

Review this guide from time to time. After being free of cigarettes for a few weeks, you may be tempted to stop doing the things that helped you quit. Keep this guidebook close by and reread the sections you need the most.

Smoking is not an option. If you goof and have a single puff on a cigarette, the chances are very high that you will return to regular smoking. No matter what crisis or temptation you face in the future, tell yourself that smoking is not an option. Stick by your decision to live smokefree—it is a good decision!

Quit clinics can help. For many, the support of a quit-smoking clinic is very helpful. If you are having difficulty remaining free of cigarettes, consider attending a clinic.

Many communities have QuitSmart classes. These classes are taught by health professionals who have been trained and certified by the author of this guide. Go to *www.QuitSmart.com* to find a class near you.

For other clinics, search on the internet or check your phonebook's yellow pages under "Smokers' Information and Treatment Centers." Be skeptical of programs that claim long-term (six months to one year) success rates of 70 percent or more. A 50 percent success rate would be very good.

Celebrate. After six-months of freedom from tobacco, do something special. Use the hundreds of dollars that did not go up in smoke to have a party, take a trip, or buy something special just for you.

My six-month anniversary of freedom from tobacco is:

_____

(date)

To celebrate I will:

_____

_____

_____

_____

Help others. Your success may inspire others to quit. You can help them by being supportive and sharing your knowledge of the quitting process.

Your doctor, dentist, and company health nurse will be interested in knowing about your experience with the QuitSmart method. They want to help people quit—they see the illness and death caused by cigarettes every day. They can use the order form on page 94 to request information or visit *www.QuitSmart.com*.

You have accomplished much. Your success in quitting smoking may inspire you to make other healthy lifestyle changes. Healthy eating, a prudent exercise program, and routine use of seat belts soon become a part of many exsmokers' lives.

Be good to yourself and enjoy your new lifestyle!

R. H. Shigley

QuitSmart® Kit

From the Director of the Duke Stop Smoking Clinic. Over 200,000 kits are in print—a best seller in the stop-smoking market.

Guidebook
Reveals how to use the QuitSmart method to break the addiction/habit of smoking

Hypnosis CD
Fosters relaxation and helps overcome psychological dependence on cigarettes

Cigarette Substitute
A patented fake cigarette with adjustable draw

Some of the Rave Reviews

"It is hard to say which of the three kit elements I enjoyed most."

Jamie Dillon, MS, RRT
Advance for Respiratory Care Practitioners

"This kit should be purchased, studied and used by all..."

Helen Sibilano, RN, MSN
Oncology Nursing Forum

"The QuitSmart Stop Smoking Kit is easy to use, interactive and informative... I enthusiastically recommend the kit."

Dr. Crystal Dunlevy
Respiratory Care

ORDER FORM

Qty		Price
___	**QuitSmart Kit**—Guidebook, Hypnosis CD, and Cigarette Substitute ($31.99 each kit)	_____
___	**QuitSmart Guidebook** ($11.99)	_____
___	**QuitSmart Hypnosis CD** ($13.99)	_____
___	**Cigarette Substitute** ($6.99)	_____
	North Carolinians add 7.0% sales tax	_____

Shipping: Add $6.00 for the first item or kit, plus 50¢ for each additional item _____

Total _____

Your Address (No PO Boxes)

Name _____

Address _____

City _____

State _____ Zip _____

Phone or e-mail _____
(In case we need to contact you about your order)

Payment Method

❏ Check to QuitSmart   ❏ MasterCard   ❏ VISA

Acct # _____ Exp. _____

Order By

Phone	*888-737-6278*
Fax	919-644-0736
Web	www.QuitSmart.com
Mail	QuitSmart, Inc. P. O. Box 99016, Duke Station Durham, NC 27708-9016

Guarantee: You may return any item within 30 days for a full refund if not satisfied

❏ Please send information on QuitSmart Leader Certification Seminars for health professionals